COMPETENCIES FOR ADVANCED PRACTICE HOSPICE AND PALLIATIVE CARE NURSES

Hospice and Palliative Nurses Association

KENDALL/HUNT PUBLISHING COMPANY
4050 Westmark Drive Dubuque, Iowa 52002

The development of these Competencies was made possible in part by a grant received by New York University from The Project Death in America.

ISBN 978-0-7872-9193-8

Printed in the United States of America
10 9 8 7 6 5 4 3 2

Advanced Practice Competency Team Members

Deborah Sherman, PhD, RN, CS, ANP
Program Coordinator, Advanced Practice/Palliative Care Master's Program
New York University
New York, NY

Patsy Abbott, RN, BSN, CHPN
Academic Liaison
The Hospice of the Florida Suncoast
Largo, FL

Michael Ryan, MS, RN
Nurse Educator
Hospice and Palliative Services
Carondelet Health Network
Tucson, AZ

Constance Dahlin, MSN, RN, CS, ANP, CHPN
Advanced Practice Palliative Care Nurse
Massachusetts General Hospital
Boston, MA

Denice Kopchak Sheehan, MSN, RN
Coordinator Palliative Care Program
Ursuline College
Cleveland Heights, OH

Susan Derby, RN, MA, CGNP
Nurse Practitioner on Pain and Palliative Care Service
Memorial Sloan-Kettering Cancer Center
New York, NY

Competency Content Reviewers

Clare Conner, PhD(c), RN
University of Vermont
North Ferrisburg, VT

Constance Dahlin, MSN, RN, CS, ANP, CHPN
Advanced Practice Palliative Care Nurse
Massachusetts General Hospital
Boston, MA

Pam Fordham, RN, DSN, FNP-C
University of Alabama
Springville, AL

Linda Gorman, MN, RN, CS, OCN, CHPN
Palliative/Hospice Clinical Nurse Specialist
Cedars/Sinai Medical Center
Los Angeles, CA

Jane Marie Kirschling, RN, DNS
Professor and Dean
University of Southern Maine
Portland, ME

Susan Riddell, MS, RN, NHA, CRNH
Administrator
Mariner Health Care
Palm City, FL

Joyce Zerwekh, RN, EdD
Florida Atlantic University
Boca Raton, FL

CONTENTS

FOREWORD

Since its inception in 1986, the Hospice and Palliative Nurses Association (HPNA) has recognized the need for methods of ensuring that the highest quality hospice and palliative care is provided to patients and families at the end of life. The National Board for Certification of Hospice and Palliative Nurses, which develops and administers the national certifying examination, was an outgrowth of the membership association adding a quality component to practice. HPNA published the first "Standards of Hospice Nursing Practice" in 1995 which were revised and expanded in 2000 and retitled "Statement on the Scope and Standards of Hospice and Palliative Practice."

COMPETENCIES

Competencies represent the quantifiable knowledge, attitudes, and skills the advanced practice hospice and palliative nurse demonstrates in the performance of safe, consistent, compassionate, state-of-the-art evidence-based end-of-life care which conforms to the patients' and their families wishes.

The use of standards, competencies and the process of accreditation are necessary and important strategies to meet stated goals. Identifying the intellectual, interpersonal, technical and moral competencies needed to practice quality end-of-life care will help to ensure these standards are met. These competencies need to be outcome-specific and measurable. Identified competencies will be the benchmark to make explicit the areas of knowledge and skills an advanced practice hospice and palliative nurse needs in order to provide quality hospice and palliative care.

Modified from the Foreword of the Professional Competencies for the Generalists Hospice and Palliative Nurse as written by Marty Ayers, PhD. (2001)

Judy Lentz, RN, MSN, OCN, NHA
Executive Director
Hospice and Palliative Nurses Association

INTRODUCTION

After reviewing and debating a number of unifying models, the generalists competency project panel utilized components of the American Association of Critical Care Nurses (AACN) Synergy Model as its framework. A core concept of this model is that characteristics of patients and families influence and drive the characteristics and competencies of nurses who oversee the care provided by nursing assistants.

The core characteristics or competencies of hospice and palliative nurses as agreed upon by this project panel include:

Clinical Judgement
Advocacy & Ethics
Professionalism
Collaboration
Systems Thinking
Cultural Competence
Facilitation of Learning
Communication
Research

DEFINITION OF COMPETENCY

The project panel used the following definition of competency to guide their work.

Competencies represent the quantifiable knowledge, attitudes, and skills that advanced practice hospice and palliative nurses demonstrate in the performance of safe, consistent, compassionate, state-of-the-art, evidence-based end-of-life care which conforms to the patients' and their families' wishes.

ADVANCED PRACTICE HOSPICE AND PALLIATIVE CARE NURSING COMPETENCIES

The advanced practice hospice and palliative care nurse is an emerging role in response to individual, professional, and societal needs related to the experience of life-limiting, progressive illness. Palliative care is defined as the management of patients with active, progressive, advanced disease for whom the prognosis is limited and focus is on care for symptom management to enhance quality of life. Advanced practice hospice and palliative care nurses exercise a high degree of critical thinking, analysis, and independent judgment, within the framework of autonomous and/or collaborative interdisciplinary practice. The Advanced Practice Hospice and Palliative Care Nurse (APHPCN) is a registered nurse (RN) who is educationally prepared at the master's level or higher in nursing as a Clinical Nurse Specialist (CNS) or Nurse Practitioner (NP). An advanced practice hospice and palliative care nurse has the knowledge, attitudes, and skills to perform all aspects of basic palliative care nursing. The APHPCN is distinguished by his/her ability to synthesize complex data, implement advanced plans of care, and provide leadership in palliative care. The roles of the advanced practice hospice and palliative care nurse include, but are not limited to: expert clinician, leader/facilitator of interdisciplinary teams, educator, researcher, consultant, collaborator, advocate, and/or administrator. The APHPCN who has fulfilled the requirements established by their state nurse practice acts may be authorized to assume autonomous responsibility for clinical role functions which may include prescription of controlled substances, medications, or therapies. The APHPCN may bill for services provided at the advanced practice level. To practice as an APHPCN, national certification in advanced practice hospice and palliative care nursing is recommended, although it is recognized that the APHPCN must have concurrent advanced practice certification in another specialty.

Advanced core competencies represent the knowledge, skills and attitudes advanced practice hospice and palliative care nurses demonstrate when providing evidence-based physical, psychosocial, emotional and spiritual/existential care to patients and families experiencing life-limiting, progressive illness. These statements further expand the core competencies of the hospice and palliative care nurse practicing at the generalist level. Care is provided in a collaborative manner, across the life span, in diverse settings, to patients and families experiencing life-limiting progressive illness. By virtue of graduate education and related clinical expertise, the advanced practice hospice and palliative care nurse demonstrates greater depth and breadth of knowledge, skills, theory, research and practice reflected in each of the following advanced practice hospice and palliative care nursing competencies.

Clinical Judgment: Advanced General Statement

Demonstrates advanced clinical judgment and decision making, based on expert knowledge and skill in the assessment, diagnosis, planning, and management of complex human responses to life-limiting, progressive illness.

Clinical Judgment: Advanced Core Competencies

Conducts comprehensive and/or problem focused physical, emotional, social, cultural, and spiritual assessments, including the multidimensional assessment of pain and other symptoms, of patients and families experiencing life-limiting, progressive illness.

Orders, may perform, and interprets common screening and diagnostic tests based on the goals of care for palliative care patients.

Analyzes and interprets history, presenting symptoms, physical findings and diagnostic information to formulate appropriate differential diagnoses for patient and families experiencing life-limiting progressive illness.

Utilizes advanced knowledge and skill to assess physical, emotional, psychosocial, and spiritual/existential suffering of patients and families experiencing life-limiting, progressive illness.

Prioritizes health problems of patients and families experiencing life-limiting, progressive illness, based on mutually derived goals of care.

Identifies expected outcomes based on critical analysis of both complex assessment data and diagnoses which are relevant to the patient, family and interdisciplinary/health care team and with consideration of risks, benefits, burden, and cost.

Applies relevant conceptual models, theories, and research in developing, implementing and evaluating comprehensive, effective, compassionate, and culturally and spiritually sensitive plans of care across a variety of health care settings which promote health and manage life-limiting, progressive illness experienced by patients and families.

Prescribes/recommends medications to alleviate pain and other symptoms associated with life-limiting, progressive illness. Manages complex pain/symptoms utilizing research-based practice.

Manages and treats complex physical, emotional, social, and spiritual problems/needs of patients and families experiencing life-limiting progressive illness by integrating appropriate non-pharmacologic and complementary/alternative therapies into the plan of care.

Provides guidance and counseling to patients and families regarding the management of life-limiting, progressive illness throughout the illness trajectory from time of diagnosis with advanced disease and into the bereavement period for families/survivors.

Assumes responsibility for the overall evaluation, documentation, and communication of care to enhance continuity of palliative care across health care settings.

Accurately documents comprehensive or problem focused palliative care of patients and families experiencing life-limiting, progressive illness, which allows for maximum reimbursement of services.

Evaluates patients' and families' responses to palliative care and the effectiveness of care in achieving palliative care outcomes, such as quality of life of patients and families

Uses palliative care outcome data to revise the individualized plan of care for patients and families and improve quality of health within the health care delivery system.

ADVOCACY AND ETHICS: ADVANCED GENERAL STATEMENT

Incorporates ethical principles and advanced practice professional standards in the care of patients and families receiving palliative care, while advocating for patients' and families' rights and access to quality palliative care.

Advocacy and Ethics: Advanced Core Competencies

Advocates for effective pain and symptom management for patients and families.

Develops, implements, and evaluates strategies to overcome patient, clinician, health care system, social, legal, or economic barriers to pain and symptom management.

Advocates for accessing quality palliative care for individuals and families including underserved and/or vulnerable populations.

Advocates for and protects patients' and families' rights, particularly with regard to end of life decision making.

Influences professional and health related outcomes in palliative care in organizational, legislative, and policy settings.

Develops, implements, and evaluates the institutional policies related to the provision of palliative care.

Participates in efforts to minimize cost and unnecessary duplication of testing and other diagnostic activities in accordance with the goals of care.

Applies theory and analysis to moral and ethical problems in health care and utilizes resources in the resolution of ethical dilemmas.

Incorporates ethical principles, advanced practice professional standards, and codes of ethics in hospice and palliative care nursing.

Emphasizes to nursing colleagues the importance of the ANA Code of Ethics and other professional position statements related to advanced practice hospice and palliative care nursing.

Assists nursing and other colleagues when faced with moral distress or ethical dilemmas in palliative care.

Demonstrates ethical conduct in palliative care practice, thereby role modeling such conduct/behavior for nursing colleagues or other health professionals.

PROFESSIONALISM: ADVANCED GENERAL STATEMENT

Demonstrates knowledge, skills, and attitudes that are consistent with the advanced Scope and Standards of Hospice and Palliative Nursing Practice *and* ANA Code of Ethics for Nurses.

Professionalism: Advanced Core Competencies

Demonstrates leadership in palliative care related to the roles of teacher, clinician, researcher, advocate, consultant, collaborator, administrator, coordinator, case manager, and leader.

Participates in practice, education, and research related to advancement of hospice and palliative care nursing.

Advocates for the role of the advanced practice hospice and palliative care nurse within the clinical setting, the community, and to the public, legislators, policy makers, and other health care professions.

Incorporates professional and legal standards into palliative care practice.

Develops evidence-based practice standards, protocols, policies, and other documents based on synthesis of scientific literature related to identified clinical problems and expected outcomes in palliative care.

Promotes physical, social, emotional, and spiritual care of self and other colleagues in palliative care.

Participates in legislative and policy-making activities which influence advanced hospice and palliative care nursing practice and the provision of quality palliative care.

Assumes accountability for hospice and palliative care nursing practice, striving to attain the highest standards of palliative care.

Evaluates own practice and the practice of subordinates in palliative care with regard to institutional, state, and federal laws and regulations, as well as patient, family, community, and environmental outcomes related to the potential or actual process and treatments.

Identifies areas of strength and areas for further development; modifies palliative care practice in response to this evaluation; obtains necessary education and/or assistance to meet learning/performance goals and improve one's palliative care practice.

Utilizes current research and scientific findings and participates in ongoing educational activities to expand advanced clinical knowledge and to enhance role performance.

Maintains expected certification, and licensure requirements in accordance with institutional, state, and federal laws and regulations, as well as the requirements of specialty nursing certification organizations.

Participates in appraisal of peer performance in palliative care to further strengthen overall palliative care team performance and effectiveness, as well communicating areas of concern to peers and/or appropriate management personnel for further action.

Contributes to the professional development and education of others to improve patient, family, community, and environmental outcomes as well as to improve her or his professional growth, especially in the areas of advanced practice hospice and palliative care nursing.

Actively participates in professional and specialty nursing organizations related to palliative care.

Publishes and shares knowledge through presentations at professional meetings to contribute to advanced practice hospice and palliative care nursing.

Serves as a role model, preceptor, mentor, and facilitator of learning in palliative care nursing and advanced practice hospice and palliative care nursing.

Contributes to the identification of future educational and research ideas, as well as to the development of creative and innovative ways for advanced practice hospice and palliative care nursing to improve care delivery and outcomes.

Serves as a liaison to institutional, local, state, and national legislative bodies to be influential regarding issues relating to advanced practice hospice and palliative care nursing with the goal of improved outcomes for the patient, family, community, and environment related to the potential or actual disease process and treatments.

COLLABORATION: ADVANCED GENERAL STATEMENT

Promotes an interdisciplinary/health care team approach to providing advanced hospice and palliative care nursing to the patient, family, community, and environment related to the potential or actual disease process and treatments.

Collaboration: Advanced Core Competencies

Creates a climate of trust and partnership with patients, families, and members of the interdisciplinary palliative care team.

Develops, implements and evaluates strategies to collaborate effectively with members of the palliative care team through the use of appropriate team building skills and consultation and recognizing each member's unique expertise and contributions.

Collaboratively assesses, plans, implements, and evaluates palliative care with other health care professionals.

Consults with other disciplines and members of the interdisciplinary palliative care team to maximize advanced hospice and palliative care nursing as related to health education, health promotion, health restoration, and/or health maintenance.

Collaborates with other members of interdisciplinary team in conducting patient/family conferences to identify goals and plans of care.

Collaborates with other disciplines and members of the interdisciplinary palliative care team regarding continuity of care, rehabilitation, and home care.

Coordinates interdisciplinary palliative care team efforts to execute comprehensive pain and symptom management.

Collaborates with other health professionals to insure access to health care and available resources are fairly distributed across patient/family populations.

Assumes leadership roles in organizing, implementing, and evaluating palliative care initiatives.

Identifies needs and obtains appropriate referrals for patients and families within a palliative care context.

Systems Thinking: Advanced General Statement

Manages and negotiates the health care delivery system to enhance quality of life for patients and families experiencing life-limiting, progressive illness and facilitate the provision of comprehensive, coordinated care within and across health care settings.

Systems Thinking: Advanced Core Competencies

Analyzes the impact of caring for individuals with life-threatening, progressive illness on family, community, and health care systems, including identification of available resources and potential barriers across all health care settings.

Utilizes systematic methods to assess the palliative care needs of patients and families.

Maintains current knowledge of the health care organization, financing of the health care system, and current trends within health care as it affects the delivery of palliative care.

Identifies the most appropriate setting for the delivery of palliative care consistent with the goals, preferences, and needs of patients and families experiencing life-limiting, progressive illness.

Provides cost effective, quality palliative care by using the most appropriate resources and delegating care to the most appropriate, qualified health care clinician.

Negotiates for palliative care services and additional specialized services with patient, family and appropriate system's agencies through case management.

Identifies, implements, and evaluates strategies to initiate and develop palliative care programs across diverse health care settings and within the context of integrated palliative care services.

Enhances the abilities of others to effect change in the health care system, based on the application of theory, recognition of mutual respect, and delineated role responsibilities, as well as facilitating the communication of palliative care recommendations.

Considers access, cost, efficacy, and quality when making palliative care decisions.

Participates in the development of institutional and health care systems policies that support quality palliative care.

Initiates and participates in continuous quality improvement efforts to evaluate the effectiveness of palliative care.

Uses information systems to support decision making and the improvement of palliative care.

Utilizes business and management strategies to provide quality palliative care and the efficient use of resources.

Participates in legislative and policy making activities that influence advanced practice hospice and palliative care nursing.

Evaluates implications of contemporary health policy on health care providers and patients and families experiencing life-limiting, progressive illness.

Cultural and Spiritual Competence: Advanced General Statement

Demonstrates and promotes culturally and spiritually competent care by respecting diversity, regarding culture, spirituality, gender, socioeconomic status, sexual orientation consistent with the advanced Scope and Standards of Hospice and Palliative Nursing Practice *and* ANA Code of Ethics for Nurses.

Cultural and Spiritual Competence: Advanced Core Competencies

Acknowledges personal values and biases and prevents these from interfering with the delivery of quality palliative care.

Assess the influences of culture and spiritual beliefs of palliative care patients and families on their health care beliefs, behaviors, practices, learning experience, and goals of care.

Acknowledges the variances in physiological and psychological responses within cultural, spiritual, racial, ethnic, age, and gender groups that may influence the development of plan of care for palliative care patients and families.

Develops, implements, and evaluates a comprehensive plan of care which reflects the cultural and spiritual values, needs, and expectations of palliative care patients and families.

Accesses appropriate resources to deliver palliative care to patients and families from other cultures.

Addresses conflicts of patients, families, and health care providers that result from differences in cultural and spiritual perspectives related to palliative care.

Educates health care providers and models culturally and spiritually competent care.

Advocates for organizational and health care systems policies that are culturally sensitive for patient and families experiencing life-limiting, progressive illness.

FACILITATOR OF LEARNING: ADVANCED GENERAL STATEMENT

Demonstrates knowledge, skills, confidence, and the application of adult learning principles when providing palliative care education to patients/families, health care professionals, and the community.

Facilitator of Learning: Advanced Core Competencies

Assesses the ongoing and changing needs of palliative care patients and families for teaching based on anticipatory guidance, care management that requires specific information or skills, and patient's understanding of his/her health and/or illness.

Creates an environment in which effective learning can take place taking into account information about cultural influences.

Employs complex strategies, interventions, and teaching methodologies based on the assessment of risks, learning theory, epidemiologic principles, and patients' and families health beliefs and practices within the context of palliative care.

Develops, implements, and evaluates formal and informal education and training in palliative care for patients, families, health care professionals and the community.

Initiates education which will influence individual and societal attitudes regarding palliative care.

Incorporates theory and research in the development, implementation and evaluation of educational offerings related to palliative care.

Disseminates state of the art palliative care knowledge at the local, state and national levels.

Communication: Advanced General Statement

Communicates effectively with palliative care patients, families, and health care professionals by applying knowledge of communication theory and principles.

Communication: Advanced Core Competencies

Monitors and reflects on own emotional response to interaction with patient and families experiencing life-limiting, progressive illness, using this knowledge to further therapeutic communication.

Creates an environment of effective and compassionate communication for palliative care patients, families, health care professionals and community.

Communicates a sense of "being present" with the patient and family experiencing life-limiting, progressive illness, providing comfort and emotional support.

Demonstrates effective communication and problem solving in complex palliative care decisions for patients, families, health care professionals and community.

Elicits information about the palliative care patient's interpretation of their health condition.

Communicates health advice, instruction, and counseling, appropriately using evidence-based rationales for patients and families experiencing life-limiting, progressive illness.

Communicates treatment options, benefits and burdens, and preferences effectively to patients, families and health care professionals in palliative care.

Facilitates conflict resolution for palliative care patients, families, and health care professionals utilizing appropriate theory and concepts.

Maintains confidentiality, while communicating data, plans and results in a manner that preserves the privacy and dignity of the palliative care patient and family.

Communicates the palliative care patients' and families' health status using appropriate terminology, format, and technology.

Evaluates knowledge and information derived from electronic and scientific information technologies as it relates to palliative care.

RESEARCH: ADVANCED GENERAL STATEMENT

Utilizes research to identify, examine, validate, and evaluate current theories and palliative care practice with the goal of improved outcomes for palliative care patients, families and the community.

Research: Advanced Core Competencies

Accesses current and relevant data needed to answer questions related to palliative care.

Initiates inquiry into comprehensive databases in order to utilize available research related to palliative care and support evidence-based practice.

Utilizes information systems for the storage and retrieval of data related to patients and families experiencing life-limiting, progressive illness.

Applies state of the art knowledge to analyze the outcomes, initiate change, and improve palliative care practice.

Evaluates the quality of research, clinical articles, Internet or web-based information related to palliative care.

Participates in or conducts research related to palliative care.